STRATEGIES FOR STRESS REDUCTION AND MENTAL WELLBEING FOR SENIORS

"Aging Gracefully, Living Mindfully: Proven Strategies for Seniors' Stress Reduction and Mental Resilience"

BLESS P. WALTON

TABLE OF CONTENTS

CHAPTER 1 6

UNDERSTANDING THE IMPACT OF AGING ON MENTAL WELLBEING 6

1.1 The Psychological Dimensions of Aging 7

1.2 Common Stressors Faced by Seniors 8

1.3 Recognizing the Importance of Mental Resilience in the Aging Process 10

CHAPTER 2 14

MINDFUL LIVING FOR SENIORS 14

2.1 Introduction to Mindfulness Practices 14

2.2 Mindful Breathing and Meditation Techniques 16

2.3 Integrating Mindfulness into Daily Activities 18

CHAPTER 3 21

PHYSICAL WELLNESS AND STRESS REDUCTION 21

3.1 The Interconnection of Physical and Mental Health 21

3.2 Exercise and its Positive Impact on Seniors' Mental Wellbeing 23

3.3 Tailoring Physical Activities to Individual Needs and Abilities 25

CHAPTER 4 29

SOCIAL CONNECTIONS AND EMOTIONAL SUPPORT 29

4.1 The Role of Social Relationships in Senior Mental Health 29

4.2 Building and Maintaining Meaningful Connections 30

4.3 Recognizing and Addressing Social Isolation 32

CHAPTER 5 36

PRACTICAL STRATEGIES FOR DAILY STRESS MANAGEMENT 36

5.1 Developing Effective Coping Mechanisms 36

5.2 Time Management and Prioritization for Seniors... 38

5.3 Creating a Holistic Daily Routine for Stress Reduction 40

CHAPTER 1

UNDERSTANDING THE IMPACT OF AGING ON MENTAL WELLBEING

As individuals transition into their golden years, it becomes increasingly important to explore the psychological dimensions of aging and the profound impact it can have on mental wellbeing. Aging is a natural and inevitable part of life, accompanied by a complex interplay of physical, emotional, and cognitive changes.

This chapter delves into the intricacies of the psychological aspects of aging, shedding light on common stressors faced by seniors and emphasizing the critical role of mental resilience in navigating the challenges associated with growing older.

1.1 The Psychological Dimensions of Aging

Aging is a multifaceted process that extends beyond the physical realm, encompassing various psychological dimensions. One of the key aspects is the evolving sense of identity and self-concept. As individuals age, they may grapple with a shifting perception of themselves, influenced by factors such as retirement, changing roles within the family, and the potential loss of independence. Exploring and understanding these shifts is crucial for maintaining a positive mental outlook.

Another psychological dimension involves cognitive changes, including alterations in memory, attention, and processing speed. While these changes are a natural part of aging, they can contribute to feelings of frustration and vulnerability. Understanding the normalcy of cognitive changes helps seniors and their caregivers navigate these transitions with patience and acceptance.

Moreover, the emotional landscape of aging is marked by a spectrum of experiences. Seniors may confront the loss of loved ones, health challenges, and a sense of isolation. Emotional resilience becomes a vital tool in coping with these changes, enabling individuals to adapt and find fulfillment despite the inevitable trials that come with aging.

1.2 Common Stressors Faced by Seniors

Aging is often accompanied by a set of common stressors that can significantly impact mental wellbeing. Financial concerns, especially in the context of retirement, can create anxiety and uncertainty. Seniors may find themselves navigating fixed incomes, rising healthcare costs, and the need to manage their resources wisely. Addressing financial stress is not just about practical solutions but also about fostering a mindset that promotes financial security and peace of mind.

Health-related stressors are another prevalent aspect of aging. Chronic illnesses, diminished physical abilities, and the potential for increased medical interventions can contribute to feelings of vulnerability. Seniors may grapple with concerns about their health, leading to anxiety and a sense of loss. It is crucial to adopt a holistic approach to health that encompasses physical, mental, and emotional well-being to mitigate the impact of these stressors.

Social factors also play a significant role in the stress experienced by seniors. The loss of friends or a spouse, coupled with changes in family dynamics, can contribute to feelings of loneliness and isolation. Maintaining and cultivating social connections becomes paramount in mitigating these stressors. Recognizing the value of relationships and actively engaging with social networks can foster a sense of belonging and emotional support.

1.3 Recognizing the Importance of Mental Resilience in the Aging Process

In the face of the psychological dimensions and common stressors associated with aging, the cultivation of mental resilience emerges as a fundamental component of positive mental wellbeing for seniors. Mental resilience involves the ability to adapt to challenges, bounce back from adversity, and maintain a sense of purpose and optimism.

One key element of mental resilience is the development of coping strategies. Seniors can benefit from identifying and adopting effective coping mechanisms that align with their individual preferences and needs. This might include practicing mindfulness, engaging in hobbies, or seeking support from friends and family. By proactively addressing stressors, seniors can enhance their capacity to navigate the complexities of aging with grace and composure.

Another aspect of mental resilience is fostering a positive mindset. Cultivating gratitude, embracing a sense of humor, and focusing on the present moment can contribute to a more optimistic outlook on life. Seniors can learn to reframe negative thoughts and perceptions, fostering a mental environment that supports their overall well-being.

Moreover, maintaining a sense of purpose and engagement in meaningful activities is vital for mental resilience. Whether through volunteer work, pursuing hobbies, or spending time with loved ones, having a sense of purpose provides a motivational anchor that can help seniors navigate the challenges of aging with a greater sense of fulfillment.

In conclusion, understanding the psychological dimensions of aging, recognizing common stressors, and prioritizing mental resilience are essential components of promoting mental wellbeing for seniors. By exploring the intricacies of the aging process and adopting proactive strategies, seniors can embrace their later years with a positive mindset, resilience, and a deep sense of fulfillment.

This foundational understanding sets the stage for the subsequent chapters, which will delve into specific strategies and practices aimed at stress reduction and mental resilience for seniors.

CHAPTER 2
MINDFUL LIVING FOR SENIORS

2.1 Introduction to Mindfulness Practices

Mindfulness, rooted in ancient contemplative traditions, has gained significant recognition in recent years for its positive impact on mental wellbeing. For seniors navigating the complexities of aging, incorporating mindfulness practices into daily life can be a transformative journey. This chapter introduces the concept of mindfulness and explores its relevance in promoting mental resilience among seniors.

Mindfulness, at its core, involves cultivating a heightened awareness of the present moment without judgment. It encourages individuals to observe their thoughts and feelings with curiosity, fostering a sense of clarity and calmness. For seniors, mindfulness offers a powerful tool to navigate the challenges of aging, promoting a positive mindset and enhancing overall mental wellbeing.

The practice of mindfulness often begins with simple techniques such as mindful breathing. By directing attention to the breath and being fully present in each inhalation and exhalation, seniors can create a sense of calm and relaxation. This introductory practice serves as a foundation for more advanced mindfulness techniques, providing an accessible entry point for those new to the practice.

2.2 Mindful Breathing and Meditation Techniques

Mindful breathing serves as a gateway to meditation, a practice that holds immense potential for seniors seeking stress reduction and mental resilience. Meditation involves intentionally directing attention inward, often through focused breathing, visualization, or mantra repetition. This section explores various meditation techniques tailored to the unique needs and abilities of seniors.

Guided meditation, where individuals follow verbal instructions to visualize calming scenes or engage in body scan exercises, can be particularly beneficial for seniors. This practice not only cultivates a sense of relaxation but also enhances self-awareness. Additionally, loving-kindness meditation, which involves directing positive intentions towards oneself and others, fosters a sense of connection and compassion, mitigating feelings of isolation that seniors may experience.

Yoga, a mind-body practice that combines physical postures, breath control, and meditation, is another valuable avenue for seniors to explore mindfulness. Modified yoga poses that accommodate physical limitations can improve flexibility, balance, and overall well-being. The integration of mindfulness into yoga sessions enhances the mind-body connection, promoting a holistic approach to health for seniors.

Breath awareness meditation, where individuals focus on the natural rhythm of their breath, serves as an adaptable and accessible practice for seniors. This technique can be practiced in various settings, making it a versatile tool for stress reduction. As seniors become more adept at directing their attention to the present moment, they develop a heightened sense of mindfulness that transcends the meditation session and permeates daily life.

2.3 Integrating Mindfulness into Daily Activities

Beyond formal meditation sessions, the integration of mindfulness into daily activities empowers seniors to live mindfully throughout their day. Mindful eating, for example, involves savoring each bite, appreciating the flavors and textures of food, and cultivating a heightened awareness of the act of nourishing the body. This practice not only contributes to physical health but also fosters a mindful approach to daily rituals.

Mindful walking is another accessible practice for seniors, promoting physical activity while enhancing awareness. Whether strolling in nature or within the confines of a living space, paying attention to each step and the surrounding environment engages the senses and facilitates a sense of presence. This practice is particularly beneficial for seniors with mobility challenges, offering a gentle yet effective way to incorporate mindfulness into their routine.

The cultivation of mindfulness can extend to activities such as gardening, art, or listening to music. Engaging in these pursuits with full attention and a non-judgmental mindset allows seniors to experience a sense of joy and fulfillment. Mindfulness becomes a companion in daily life, offering support in navigating both routine and unexpected moments with grace and equanimity.

In conclusion, mindfulness practices provide seniors with valuable tools for stress reduction and mental resilience. From the foundational practice of mindful breathing to the exploration of meditation techniques and the integration of mindfulness into daily activities, seniors can embark on a journey that enhances their overall mental wellbeing.

This chapter sets the stage for the subsequent chapters, which will delve into physical wellness, social connections, and practical strategies for daily stress management in the pursuit of aging gracefully and living mindfully.

CHAPTER 3

PHYSICAL WELLNESS AND STRESS REDUCTION

3.1 The Interconnection of Physical and Mental Health

The symbiotic relationship between physical and mental health is a fundamental aspect of overall wellbeing, especially for seniors navigating the aging process. This chapter explores the interconnected nature of physical and mental health and emphasizes the role of physical wellness in stress reduction.

Physical activity has a profound impact on mental health, influencing neurotransmitter release, reducing inflammation, and promoting the growth of new neurons. For seniors, maintaining an active lifestyle is not only beneficial for physical health but also plays a crucial role in supporting cognitive function and emotional wellbeing. Recognizing this interconnection lays the foundation for a holistic approach to stress reduction and mental resilience.

A sedentary lifestyle can contribute to feelings of lethargy and negatively impact mood. Conversely, engaging in regular physical activity releases endorphins, the body's natural mood enhancers. The stimulation of the brain during exercise helps mitigate symptoms of anxiety and depression, common concerns for seniors. By understanding the reciprocal relationship between physical and mental health, seniors can make informed choices that promote overall wellness.

3.2 Exercise and its Positive Impact on Seniors' Mental Wellbeing

Exercise stands out as a powerful tool for stress reduction and mental wellbeing among seniors. The benefits extend beyond the physical realm, encompassing cognitive function, emotional balance, and social engagement. This section explores the positive impact of exercise on seniors' mental health and suggests various forms of physical activity tailored to their unique needs.

Aerobic exercise, such as walking, swimming, or cycling, has been shown to enhance cognitive function and reduce the risk of cognitive decline in seniors. The increased blood flow to the brain during aerobic activity supports the growth of new neurons and strengthens neural connections.

As a result, seniors who engage in regular aerobic exercise often experience improved memory, attention, and overall cognitive performance.

Strength training, focusing on resistance exercises for major muscle groups, contributes to physical resilience and functional independence. Beyond its physical benefits, strength training boosts self-esteem and fosters a sense of accomplishment, positively influencing mental wellbeing.

Seniors can explore activities like weightlifting, resistance band exercises, or bodyweight workouts to enhance both physical and mental strength.

Mind-body exercises, including yoga and tai chi, offer a holistic approach to physical and mental wellness. These practices combine gentle movements with mindfulness, promoting relaxation, flexibility, and stress reduction. Seniors can benefit from the meditative aspects of these activities, which contribute to a calm and focused mind, reducing the impact of stressors on mental health.

3.3 Tailoring Physical Activities to Individual Needs and Abilities

Recognizing the diversity of seniors' abilities and health conditions, it is essential to tailor physical activities to meet individual needs. This customization ensures that each senior can engage in exercises that align with their physical capabilities, making physical wellness accessible and enjoyable for everyone.

Low-impact exercises, such as water aerobics or stationary biking, provide a gentle yet effective way for seniors with joint concerns or mobility limitations to stay active. These activities reduce the risk of injury while still offering cardiovascular benefits and stress reduction.

Group activities, such as dance classes or walking clubs, foster social connections alongside physical exercise. The social component is particularly valuable for seniors, as it enhances a sense of community and combats feelings of isolation. Combining physical activity with social engagement creates a holistic approach to wellbeing, addressing both the physical and mental aspects of health.

In-home exercises, including chair exercises and gentle stretching routines, cater to seniors who prefer or require a more accessible approach to physical activity. These routines can be adapted to accommodate varying levels of mobility, allowing seniors to engage in regular exercise within the comfort of their homes.

In conclusion, the interconnection of physical and mental health underscores the importance of physical wellness in stress reduction for seniors. Exercise, in its various forms, emerges as a key strategy for promoting mental resilience and overall wellbeing.

By tailoring physical activities to individual needs and abilities, seniors can embark on a personalized journey towards enhanced physical and mental health. This chapter sets the stage for the subsequent exploration of social connections and practical strategies for daily stress management in the pursuit of aging gracefully and living mindfully.

CHAPTER 4

SOCIAL CONNECTIONS AND EMOTIONAL SUPPORT

4.1 The Role of Social Relationships in Senior Mental Health

The significance of social connections in influencing mental health is a well-established aspect of human well-being, and this holds especially true for seniors. As individuals age, the quality and quantity of their social relationships play a pivotal role in shaping mental resilience and overall emotional wellness.

This chapter explores the profound impact of social relationships on senior mental health, emphasizing the importance of cultivating and maintaining meaningful connections.

Social interactions contribute to emotional support, companionship, and a sense of belonging—essential elements for seniors navigating the challenges of aging. Positive social relationships act as a buffer against stress, providing a support system that fosters emotional resilience.

Maintaining a robust social network is linked to various mental health benefits, including reduced feelings of loneliness, enhanced cognitive function, and a more positive outlook on life.

4.2 Building and Maintaining Meaningful Connections

Building and sustaining meaningful connections in later life involves intentional efforts to foster relationships that bring joy, understanding, and emotional support. Seniors can take proactive steps to build new connections and nurture existing ones, contributing to their overall mental and emotional wellbeing.

Community involvement is a powerful avenue for seniors to forge new connections. Joining clubs, attending social events, or participating in volunteer activities creates opportunities to meet like-minded individuals and build friendships. Shared interests provide a foundation for meaningful connections, fostering a sense of purpose and engagement.

Family ties remain a cornerstone of social relationships for seniors. Strengthening connections with family members through regular communication, shared activities, and the celebration of milestones contributes to a robust support system. Family relationships provide a sense of continuity and belonging, offering emotional support during both joyful and challenging times.

Friendships, whether longstanding or newly formed, are vital for seniors seeking companionship and emotional connection. Cultivating friendships involves investing time and effort in shared activities, communication, and mutual support. Quality relationships contribute to a sense of fulfillment and provide a valuable network for coping with life's ups and downs.

4.3 Recognizing and Addressing Social Isolation

Social isolation, characterized by a lack of meaningful social connections, is a prevalent concern for seniors and poses a significant threat to mental health. Recognizing the signs of social isolation and taking proactive steps to address this issue are crucial for promoting emotional wellbeing among seniors.

Common signs of social isolation include withdrawal from social activities, a decline in communication with friends and family, and a persistent sense of loneliness. Seniors, caregivers, and community members alike can play a role in identifying and addressing these signs, offering support and resources to mitigate the impact of social isolation.

Technology can serve as a valuable tool for combating social isolation, especially in today's digital age. Seniors can explore virtual communication platforms, social media, and online communities to stay connected with friends and family. Learning to navigate these technologies opens new avenues for social interaction and reduces barriers to meaningful connections.

Community programs and support services tailored to seniors provide opportunities for social engagement. Senior centers, recreational activities, and wellness programs offer venues for meeting others and participating in shared experiences. These community resources contribute to a sense of belonging and help combat the detrimental effects of social isolation.

In conclusion, the role of social relationships in senior mental health is undeniable, with meaningful connections serving as a cornerstone of emotional wellbeing. Building and maintaining these connections require intentional efforts, but the rewards are immense—reduced feelings of loneliness, enhanced emotional resilience, and an enriched quality of life. This chapter sets the stage for the exploration of practical strategies for daily stress management, emphasizing the interconnected nature of physical, social, and mental wellbeing for seniors in their pursuit of aging gracefully and living mindfully.

CHAPTER 5
PRACTICAL STRATEGIES FOR DAILY STRESS MANAGEMENT

5.1 Developing Effective Coping Mechanisms

As seniors navigate the challenges of aging, developing effective coping mechanisms becomes a key component of daily stress management. Coping mechanisms are strategies and techniques individuals use to handle stress and adversity. This chapter explores a range of practical coping mechanisms tailored to the unique needs of seniors, empowering them to navigate life's ups and downs with resilience.

Cognitive strategies, such as reframing negative thoughts and cultivating a positive mindset, play a pivotal role in effective stress management. Seniors can learn to challenge and change unhelpful thought patterns, focusing on solutions rather than dwelling on problems. This shift in mindset contributes to a more optimistic outlook, reducing the impact of stressors on mental wellbeing.

Emotional expression is another valuable coping mechanism. Seniors can benefit from sharing their feelings with friends, family, or support groups. Whether through conversation, journaling, or creative expression, expressing emotions provides an outlet for stress and fosters a sense of connection and understanding.

Mindfulness practices, introduced in Chapter 2, serve as powerful coping mechanisms for daily stress management. Seniors can incorporate mindful breathing, meditation, or simply being present at the moment to cultivate a calm and centered mindset. These practices ease quick pressure as well as add to long-haul mental versatility.

5.2 Time Management and Prioritization for Seniors

Effective time management is crucial for seniors aiming to balance various aspects of their lives and minimize stress. Time management involves setting priorities, organizing tasks, and allocating time efficiently. Seniors can adopt strategies to optimize their time and energy, enhancing their ability to cope with stressors.

Prioritization begins with identifying and focusing on essential tasks. Seniors can categorize activities as high, medium, or low priority, allowing them to allocate time and resources effectively. By tackling high-priority tasks first, they can reduce the sense of overwhelm and maintain a sense of accomplishment.

Establishing a routine contributes to effective time management, providing structure and predictability. Seniors can create a daily schedule that incorporates essential activities such as exercise, social interactions, and relaxation. Consistency in routines promotes a sense of stability and control, reducing the potential for stress associated with uncertainty.

Setting realistic goals aligns with effective time management. Seniors can break down larger tasks into smaller, manageable steps, making progress more achievable. Celebrating small accomplishments along the way fosters a positive mindset and motivation to continue managing time effectively.

5.3 Creating a Holistic Daily Routine for Stress Reduction

A holistic daily routine encompasses various elements of physical, mental, and social wellbeing, contributing to comprehensive stress reduction. Seniors can tailor their routines to incorporate practices that address different aspects of their health and promote overall wellbeing.

Starting the day with mindful practices, such as meditation or gentle stretching, sets a positive tone for the day ahead. Mindful activities engage the senses and promote a calm mindset, providing a foundation for navigating daily stressors with resilience.

Physical activity, as discussed in Chapter 3, is a fundamental component of a holistic routine. Seniors can schedule regular exercise, adapting activities to their preferences and abilities. This may include a morning walk, a yoga session, or other forms of exercise that align with their physical health goals.

Social interactions are integral to a holistic daily routine. Seniors can incorporate time for connecting with friends, family, or community members. Whether through phone calls, in-person visits, or participation in social activities, fostering social connections contributes to emotional support and reduces feelings of isolation.

Prioritizing self-care is a key element of a holistic routine. Seniors can engage in activities that bring them joy and relaxation, whether it's reading, gardening, or pursuing hobbies. Allocating time for self-care reinforces a sense of personal fulfillment and contributes to emotional wellbeing.

In conclusion, practical strategies for daily stress management empower seniors to navigate the complexities of aging with resilience and grace.

Developing effective coping mechanisms, implementing time management strategies, and creating a holistic daily routine contribute to a comprehensive approach to stress reduction.

This chapter serves as a culmination of strategies presented throughout the book, highlighting the interconnected nature of physical, social, and mental wellbeing for seniors in their pursuit of aging gracefully and living mindfully.